METHYLENE BLUE

A deep dive into its scientific and therapeutic wonders

Frank Imeldas

copyright@2024

Chapter one
METHYLENE BLUE 3

Chapter Two
Chemical and physical properties 10

Chapter Three
Applications in the Environment and Industry 37

Chapter Four
Applications and Discoveries in Medicine ... 48

Chapter Five
The Hazards and Side Effects of Methylene Blue 88

Chapter Six
Overview of Clinical Trials 97

Chapter one

METHYLENE BLUE

Methylene blue is a synthetic chemical compound with a wide range of applications in medicine, biology, and chemistry. Here is an overview of its properties, possible uses and significance:

Chemical Properties

- **Chemical Formula**: $C_{16}H_{18}ClN_3S$
- **Molecular Weight**: 319.85 g/mol
- **Appearance**: Dark green crystalline powder that yields a blue solution when dissolved in water or alcohol.

History and Discovery of Methylene Blue

Discovery

- **Synthesis and First Discovery (1876)** German chemist Heinrich Caro produced methylene blue for the first time in 1876. Caro was employed by the large chemical business BASF at the time that the synthetic dye industry was growing. The finding was a part of a larger initiative to develop synthetic dyes in place of natural dyes, which were more expensive to make and less stable.

Early Applications in Science and Medicine

- **Medical Applications (1891)**

  In 1891, German scientist and physician Paul Ehrlich made the discovery that methylene blue had therapeutic potential. Ehrlich was able to distinguish between different kinds of cells and microorganisms by staining tissues with methylene blue. The foundation for contemporary histology and microbiology was established by this breakthrough.

  Methylene blue was first used as an antimalarial drug as a result of Ehrlich's research. His discovery that the dye could both kill the Plasmodium malaria parasite and selectively stain specifically stands as one of the first instances of targeted medication therapy.

- **In the Treatment of Methemoglobinemia**

  Methemoglobinemia, a disorder in which hemoglobin is unable to efficiently deliver oxygen to body tissues was later shown to be effectively treated with methylene blue. By acting as a reducing agent, the dye helps to return methemoglobin to its original functional form, hemoglobin. Its most important use in modern medicine is still this one.

Advancement and Widespread Application

- **Expansion to Other Health Applications**
  Methylene blue's uses in the early 1900s went beyond treating methemoglobinemia and antimalarial treatment. It was applied as a surgical and medical imaging diagnostic tool, as well as a treatment for a variety of infections.
  After the dye's antibacterial qualities were investigated, bacterial illnesses, including urinary tract infections, were treated with it.
- **Development in Scientific Research** Methylene blue

emerged as a crucial instrument in the fields of biochemistry and cell biology in particular. Its staining abilities were applied to proteins, nucleic acids, and biological structures for identification and analysis. Additionally, scientists started looking at its neuroprotective qualities and its potential for treating neurodegenerative illnesses like Parkinson's and Alzheimer's.

Modern Development

- **New Developments and Ongoing Research**

  Methylene blue has experienced a rise in interest recently because of its potential to cure a number of illnesses outside of its traditional usage. Research has concentrated on its neuroprotective effects, antioxidant capabilities, and possible role in mitochondrial function. Clinical trials are being conducted to investigate its efficacy in treating illnesses such as sepsis, cancer, and cognitive impairments.

Chapter Two
Chemical and physical properties

A comprehensive examination of the chemical composition, manufacturing processes, and physical attributes of methylene blue.

Analyzing its redox characteristics and how it interacts with biological molecules.

- **A Historical Perspective**

  A chronological narrative detailing the invention and advancement of methylene blue, encompassing its preliminary use in both industry and medicine.

Biographies of key researchers and historical milestones that influenced its current application.

- **Usage in Medicine**

  A thorough analysis of the medicinal applications of methylene blue, encompassing its function in neuroprotection, antimalarial qualities, and therapy of methemoglobinemia. Investigation of its diagnostic applications in different medical procedures and possible medical applications in the future.

- **Pharmacology and Toxicology**

  A comprehensive analysis of methylene blue's pharmacokinetics and pharmacodynamics.

A comprehensive evaluation of its safety, toxicity, and side effect profiles to offer a fair assessment of its medical uses.

- **Scientific Research and Case Studies**

Presentation of significant case studies and clinical experiments demonstrating the practical applications of methylene blue, as well as its limitations.

Examining current studies and new developments that point to potential uses for methylene blue in different contexts.

- **Industrial and Environmental Application**
  An analysis of methylene blue's applications in a range of sectors, such as environmental monitoring, biological staining, and textile coloring.
  Talk about how it affects the environment and how it biodegradation.
- **Future Directions**
  Future projections for methylene blue predicated on new scientific findings and patterns in ongoing research. Determining possible new uses and areas that require more research.

Chemical Composition and Synthesis

Chemical Structure

- **Molecular Formula and Structure Molecular Formula:** C16H18ClN3S
  IUPAC Name: 3,7-bis(dimethylamino)-phenothiazin-5-ium chloride

Overview of the structure

- Methylene blue is a dye that belongs to the phenothiazine class and is an aromatic chemical.
- Its structure is made up of two dimethylamino groups that are connected to the phenothiazine core at positions 3 and 7.

- One reason for its solubility in water is that it exists as a chloride salt.

Structure in Three Dimensions

- An explanation of methylene blue's three-dimensional structure, including bond angles and substituent placement in space.
- The structure's effect on the material's chemical and physical properties.

Electronic Characteristics

- The electron delocalization inside the phenothiazine ring structure is discussed.
- An explanation of the absorption spectrum, which

shows how the electronic structure affects the object's redox

Synthesis

- **Historical Synthesis Techniques**

  An overview of Heinrich Caro's initial synthesis from 1876. N, N-dimethylaniline is oxidized in the presence of sulfur and a weak oxidizing agent, such as sodium dichromate, in the basic process involved.

- **Modern Synthesis Methods**

  Industrial Synthesis: A detailed explanation of how large-scale industrial production is carried out.

  Important ingredients and

setups for the procedure.

Laboratory Synthesis: A thorough guide on the creation of methylene blue in the lab. Reaction conditions, equipment, and chemicals needed.

Differential Synthesis Route

Talking about different synthetic pathways that have been created over time.

Evaluation of the effectiveness, yield, and environmental effects of various techniques.

Crystallization and Purification

Purification techniques for methylene blue to get rid of contaminants and byproducts. Methods for crystallizing methylene blue to provide high-purity samples for use in research and healthcare.

Stability and Chemical Reactions

- **Redox Reactions:** Explanations of the redox indicator function of methylene blue.
  A description of its redox cycle, which consists of reduction to leucomethylene blue and then reoxidation.
- **The stability of chemicals**
  Elements influencing methylene blue's stability in different conditions (pH, light, temperature, etc.).
  Suggested storage parameters to keep things stable and stop deterioration.

- **Derivatives and Modification**

  A summary of the chemical changes and methylene blue derivatives.

  Potential advantages and uses of these compounds in medical and scientific research.

Application Originating from Chemical properties

- **Dyeing and Staining**

  An explanation of how methylene blue's chemical structure contributes to how well it works as a dye and stain. Use in biological staining methods in the textile industry.

- **Therapeutic Uses**

Explanation of how its redox characteristics help with medical conditions including neuroprotection and methemoglobinemia.

- **Applications of Scientific Research**

    The scientific fields of biochemistry, cell biology, and neuroscience employ methylene blue.

    Use as a research instrument in labs and for the study of biological processes.

Physical Properties

Appearance and Physical Qualities

- **Color and Form**: Blue crystals or a dark green crystalline powder are the usual forms of methylene blue.
  Its distinctive and clearly identifiable deep blue color is seen in aqueous solution.
- **Solubility**
  Water Solubility: Very soluble in water, creating a blue mixture.
  Its solubility in water is crucial for its use in biological staining and medicinal procedures.
  Solubility in Other Solvents: Limited solubility in non-polar

solvents such as chloroform and benzene.

Soluble in ethanol and other polar solvents.

- **Boiling and Melting Points**
  Melting Point: Approximately between 100 to 110°C (the decomposition).
  Boiling Point: Methylene blue decomposes before boiling, hence this is irrelevant.

Spectroscopic Properties

- **Spectrum of Absorption:** In the visible region, methylene blue exhibits a distinctive absorption peak.
  In aqueous solution, the maximum absorption (λmax) is

approximately 660–670 nm. Methylene blue concentrations in solutions are measured using the absorption spectrum.

- **Fluorescence:** Demonstrates fluorescence, making it suitable for a range of fluorescence microscopy techniques.

  Emission of Fluorescence peaks at 688 nm when excited at 660 nm.

- **Nuclear Magnetic Resonance (NMR) and Infrared (IR) Spectra**

  IR Spectrum: Reports on the functional groups that are present in the molecule (e.g., aromatic C-H bond peaks, C-N, and C-S peaks).

NMR Spectrum: This can be used to verify the structure since it displays the typical chemical shifts for the dimethylamino and aromatic protons.

Redox characteristics

- **Oxidation Reduction Behavior**: Methylene blue is a well-known redox indicator, alternates between its reduced (colorless) and oxidized (blue) states.

Redox Potential: About +0.53 V is the redox potential for the methylene blue/leucomethylene blue couple.

- **Role in Biological System:** Methylene blue's redox

characteristics allow it to be used in biological systems to research oxidative stress and electron transport chains.

Stability and Decomposition

- **The stability of chemicals:** Stable in normal conditions, but light and hot temperatures might cause it to become unstable.
Photodegradation, which lowers its effectiveness, can result from prolonged exposure to light.
- **Decomposition:** When heated, it breaks down and releases harmful gasses like nitrogen oxides (NOx) and sulfur oxides (SOx).
The phenothiazine ring structure

can potentially break down under conditions that are extremely basic or acidic.

Physical Interactions

- **Interaction with Biological Molecules:** It's used as a biological stain is based on its high binding to proteins and nucleic acids.

  It can be seen under a microscope due to its interactions with cellular components.

- **Aggregation Behavior:** In solution, aggregates frequently form, particularly at high concentrations.

  Aggregation may affect the substance's spectroscopic

characteristics as well as efficacy in staining and medicinal application.

Applications Associated with Physical Characteristics

- **Biological Staining:** This stain is used in histology and microbiology because of its bright color and strong affinity to cellular components. Frequently used for tasks like cell nuclei visualization and Gram staining.
- **Medical Diagnostics and Procedures:** Because of its solubility and visibility, it is used in diagnostic techniques such sentinel lymph node mapping.

Made use of its redox characteristics in medicinal treatments such as methemoglobinemia.

- **Uses in Industry:** Because of its water solubility and durability, it is used in the textile industry to dyeing fabrics.

Mechanisms of Action

Electron Transfer and Redox Properties

- **Oxidation-Reduction Behavior:** Methylene blue is a strong redox agent that can be reduced reversibly to produce the colorless leucomethylene blue.

Its medicinal and diagnostic uses depend heavily on this redox cycle.

Mechanism: Electrons are accepted by methylene blue (oxidized form) to transform it into leucomethylene blue (reduced form).
After then, leucomethylene blue can give electrons to become methylene blue again.

- **Transmission of Electrons in Biological Systems:** Methylene blue functions as an electron acceptor or donor in biological systems.

It takes part in redox reactions within the cell, impacting functions including oxidative phosphorylation and mitochondrial respiration.

Interaction with Components of the Cell

- **Attachment to Proteins and Nucleic Acids:** Methylene blue binds firmly to proteins and nucleic acids, including DNA and RNA.

  Mechanism: DNA base pairs are intercalated by the planar aromatic structure, which stabilizes the double helix and influences transcription and replication.

  Moreover, it attaches to proteins especially those involve in redox processes.

- **Mechanism of Retention:** Its application as a biological stain is supported by its binding to proteins and nucleic acids.

 Mechanism: Methylene blue preferentially attaches to negatively charged cellular components, making them visible under a microscope. It does this by intercalating with DNA to stain cell nuclei.

Antibiotic and Antiparasitic Actions

- **Antimicrobial Qualities:** Broad-spectrum antibacterial action against bacteria, fungi, and parasites is exhibited by methylene blue.

 Mechanism: Inhibits vital

enzymes and disrupts microbial cell membranes.

When exposed to light, it produces reactive oxygen species (ROS), which can cause oxidative damage.

- **Antiparasitic Action:** Potent against parasites that cause malaria (Plasmodium species).

Mechanism: Prevents the activity of heme polymerase, an enzyme essential to the survival of parasites in red blood cells. Causes oxidative stress, harming the biological components of the parasite.

Therapeutic Application

- **Methemoglobinemia Treatment**: Hemoglobin is

oxidized to methemoglobin, which is unable to bind oxygen, a condition known as hemoglobinemia.

Mechanism: NADPH-methaemoglobin reductase, an enzyme, mediates the reduction by moving electrons from NADPH to methylene blue.

> Methylene blue functions as an electron donor, converting methemoglobin back to functional hemoglobin.

- **Neuroprotective Effects:** Methylene blue's potential to protect against diseases like Parkinson's and Alzheimer's has been studied.

Mechanism: Promotes electron transfer in the electron

transport chain, which improves mitochondrial activity.
Scavenges reactive oxygen species and stabilizes the redox state of cells to reduce oxidative stress.

- **Photodynamic treatment and photosensitization:** Used in photodynamic therapy to treat specific cancers and infections.
Mechanism: Methylene blue selectively accumulates in cancer cells or contaminated tissues, making them vulnerable to light-induced harm. Methylene blue produces reactive oxygen species (ROS) upon light activation, which results in targeted cell damage and death.

Applications for Diagnosis

- **Visualization in Surgical Procedures:** When doing surgery, structures are highlighted with methylene blue.
  Mechanism: The vivid color of the dye facilitates the visualization of anatomical characteristics and the identification of issues such as leaks or blockages.
- **Sentinel Lymph Node Mapping:** This technique is employed during cancer procedures to locate sentinel lymph nodes.
  Mechanism: injected methylene blue stains sentinel

lymph nodes for simple identification and removal after passing through lymphatic vessels.

Chapter Three

Applications in the Environment and Industry

- **Environmental Monitoring:** This technique is used to identify and quantify different types of environmental pollutant.

  Mechanism: Spectroscopic measurements of the color change caused by the reaction of methylene blue with particular pollutants are possible.

- **Textile Dyeing:** Used to dye materials and fabrics.

  Mechanism: The fabric's fibers bind to the dye molecules, creating a bright and long-lasting coloration.

Early Applications in Industry and Medicine

Industrial Applications

Textile Dyeing

- **Original Use:** Shortly after Heinrich Caro synthesized it in 1876, methylene blue was one among the first synthetic dyes to be used in the textile industry.
- **Application:** Compared to natural dyes, it was more economical and consistent in giving textiles a vibrant and dependable blue color.

- **Significance:** This application aided in the expansion of the synthetic dye sector and paved the way for the creation of numerous other synthetic dyes.

Biological Staining

- **Discovery:** Methylene blue's discovery as a biological stain was identified in the late 19th century by Paul Ehrlich, a pioneering German physician and scientist.
- **Application:** Stains tissues and microorganisms to make cellular structures under a microscope visible.
- **Significance:** This use allowed scientists to distinguish between various cell and

microorganisms, laying the foundation for modern histology and microbiology.

Applications in Medicine

Antimalarial Agent

- **Early Research:** In the late 19th century, Paul Ehrlich conducted more research on the possible use of methylene blue as an antimalarial agent.
- **Application:** It was discovered that the dye could both kill and stain the Plasmodium, malaria parasite, making it one of the first examples of targeted drug therapy.
- **Significance:** This discovery demonstrated the therapeutic

potential of methylene blue and creates the path for further drug development, even if it was eventually superseded by more potent antimalarial drugs.

Methemoglobinemia Treatment

- **Identification:** Methemoglobinemia, a disorder where hemoglobin is oxidized to methemoglobin, which is unable to properly release oxygen to tissues, has been found to be effectively treated by methylene blue.
- **Application:** It functions as a reducing agent, changing methemoglobin back into hemoglobin and regaining its ability to carry oxygen.

- **Significance:** Treating methemoglobinemia patients with this medication is still one of the most important medicinal applications of methylene blue.

Use of Antimicrobials and Disinfection

- **Early Uses:** Methylene blue was used to treat a variety of infections in the early 20th century due to its antimicrobial qualities.
- **Application:** It was used as a wound dressing and in urine antiseptics to treat and prevent infections.
- **Significance:** Although the discovery of antibiotics later overshadowed methylene blue's

antimicrobial qualities, the chemical is still used in some situations, particularly where antibiotic resistance is a concern.

Diagnostic Tool

- **Surgical Applications:** During surgical procedures, methylene blue was used as a diagnostic tool to identify anatomical features and pathologies.
- **Application:** During cancer surgery, surgeons used it to identify sentinel lymph nodes, visualize the lymphatic system, and find fistulas and leaks in the gastrointestinal tract.
- **Significance:** Its application in diagnosis enhanced the

precision and results of surgical operations, rendering it a vital instrument in medical practice.

Expansion and Diversification

Scientific Research

- **Scientific Research Contributions:** Methylene blue's staining properties have made it a popular instrument in scientific research, especially in the fields of cell biology and biochemistry.
- **Application:** Methylene blue was used by researchers to study and visualize proteins, nucleic acids, and cellular structures.
- **Significance:** This led to a greater understanding of cellular

and molecular biology and enabled numerous scientific discoveries.

Neuroprotective Research

- **Initial Findings:** Research into methylene blue's neuroprotective qualities started in the early 20th century.
- **Application:** Research has shown that it may be able to treat neurodegenerative illnesses and preserve neural tissue.
- **Significance:** Research on this topic has been going strong, with studies looking into its application in ailments including Parkinson's and Alzheimer's diseases.

Research and Development Milestones

Early Discovery and Application in Industry

Heinrich Caro's synthesis (1876)

- **Milestone:** While employed at BASF, Heinrich Caro synthesized methylene blue.
- **Significance:** Methylene blue's journey as a synthetic dye began with this synthesis, which paved the way for its early use in the textile industry for fabric dyeing.

Introduction to Biological Staining (Late 19th Century)

- **Milestone:** The staining of biological tissues and microorganisms by methylene blue was discovered by Paul Ehrlich.
- **Significance:** By improving the ability to see and distinguish cellular structures under a microscope, this discovery transformed the fields of histology and microbiology.

Chapter Four

Applications and Discoveries in Medicine

Antimalarial Properties (Late 19th Century)

- **Milestone:** Paul Ehrlich's studies revealed the antimalarial potential of methylene blue.
- **Significance:** It was among the first medications used to treat malaria, indicating the potential of synthetic chemicals in the treatment of diseases.

Treatment of Methemoglobinemia (Early 20th-century)

- **Milestone:** Methylene blue was found to be an effective treatment for methemoglobinemia.

- **Significance:** By restoring hemoglobin's ability to carry oxygen, this application is still vital to medicine and can save lives.

Use of Antimicrobials (Initial 20th Century)

- **Milestone:** The antibacterial properties of methylene blue were used to treat infections.
- **Significance:** Offered a way to treat and disinfect before antibiotics were widely used.

Tools for Research and Diagnosis

Application in Diagnostic Processes (Early to Mid-20th Century)

- **Milestone:** The use of methylene blue to visualize anatomical structures during surgical diagnostic procedures.
- **Significance:** Enhanced surgical precision and results, especially in sentinel lymph node identification and gastrointestinal leak detection.

Scientific Research and Staining Methods (20th-century)

- **Milestone:** Widely used in scientific studies to stain and visualize tissues, cells, and microorganism.
- **Significance:** By using improved visualization techniques, major advancements in cell biology, biochemistry, and microbiology were made possible.

Increasing the Therapeutic Uses

Neuroprotective research (early 20th century to present)

- **Milestone:** Research into the neuroprotective qualities of methylene blue were launched, with the goal of treating neurodegenerative diseases.
- **Significance:** Research on its efficacy in ailments including Parkinson's and Alzheimer's disease is still ongoing, underscoring its potential as a therapeutic agent.

Photodynamic therapy (mid to late 20th century)

- **Milestone:** Exploring the application of methylene blue in photodynamic treatment for infections and cancer.
- **Significance:** Shown that it may produce reactive oxygen species when light is activated, which can cause specific cell damage and death and pave the way for new cancer therapy avenues.

Modern Developments and Innovations

FDA Approved for a Range of Medical Applications (late 20th to early 21st century)

- **Milestone:** FDA approval for methylene blue as a diagnostic tool and treatment for diseases such methemoglobinemia and ifosfamide-induced encephalopathy.
- **Significance:** Methylene blue's medical uses are officially recognized and regulated, guaranteeing its safe and efficient use in clinical settings.

Research on Antiviral Properties (21st Century)

- **Milestone:** Studies exploring the possible antiviral qualities of methylene blue, particularly its effectiveness against viruses such as SARS-CoV-2 and HIV.
- **Significance:** Highlighted attention to its potential for creating new antiviral therapies, strengthening the ongoing fight against viral infections.

Industrial and Environmental Innovations (21st-century)

- **Milestone:** The use of methylene blue in green chemistry and environmental monitoring.

- **Significance:** Showed its adaptability and usefulness in identifying environmental pollutants and encouraging environmentally friendly industrial practices.

Medicinal Applications of Methylene Blue

Beyond its historical and industrial usage, methylene blue has been found to have a variety of therapeutic benefits in a range of medical conditions and settings. Here are a few of its most important medicinal uses:

Methemoglobinemia Treatment

- **Mechanism:** Hemoglobin's ability to carry oxygen is

restored when methylene blue, a reducing chemical, converts ferric iron (Fe^{3+}) in methemoglobin back to ferrous iron (Fe^{2+}).

- **Indication:**
Methemoglobinemia, a disorder in which iron oxidizes to a ferric state, impairing hemoglobin's ability to release oxygen efficiently.
- **Administration:** Methylene blue is usually injected intravenously. Once inside the body, it quickly spreads to all parts of the body and acts on the methemoglobin in erythrocytes.

Ifosfamide-induced Encephalopathy

- **Mechanism:** By acting as a cofactor for monoamine oxidase (MAO), methylene blue prevents the build-up of hazardous metabolites such as chloroacetaldehyde, the neurotoxic metabolite of ifosfamide.
- **Indication:** Preventing and treating encephalopathy brought on by ifosfamide, a dangerous side effect linked to high-dose chemotherapy.
- **Administration:** To lessen or avoid neurotoxicity, intravenous administration is used either

during or after ifosfamide infusion.

Syndrome of Vasoplegia in Cardiothoracic Surgery

- **Mechanism:** Vasoplegic syndrome, which is characterized by persistent hypotension despite adequate cardiac output, can be lessened by the vasoconstrictive qualities of methylene blue.
- **Indication:** Used to enhance vascular tone and control blood pressure during or after heart surgery.
- **Administration:** To prevent side effects such as methemoglobinemia, intravenous administration of

regulated doses under medical supervision is recommended.

Agent for diagnosis

Application: Methylene blue is a diagnostic tool used in a range of medical procedures:

- **Sentinel Lymph Node Mapping:** An injection made close to a tumor helps locate sentinel lymph nodes, which helps with cancer staging and surgical planning.
- **Localization of Fistulas:** Tracks the appearance of fistulas or gastrointestinal leaks in the digestive tract.
- **Ophthalmic Surgery:** Stains tissues and membranes to help

with visualization during some eye surgeries.

Mechanism: During surgical or diagnostic procedures, anatomical features or abnormalities can be easily identified and localized thanks to the dye's vivid coloration.

Antiviral Properties (Emerging Research)

- **Mechanism:** According to recent research, methylene blue may possess antiviral qualities that could prevent viruses from replicating or infecting host cells.
- **Indication:** Investigations into its possible application against

viral diseases, such as SARS-CoV-2 and HIV, are still continuing.

- **Administration:** Although further research is needed, topical application or inhalation in the case of viral infections are two possible routes of administration.

Neuroprotective Effects (Research Area)

- **Mechanism:** By improving mitochondrial function, reducing oxidative stress, and encouraging neuronal survival, methylene blue has demonstrated potential neuroprotective effects.

- **Indication:** Investigated for potential application in neurodegenerative conditions like traumatic brain injury, Parkinson's disease, and Alzheimer's disease.
- **Administration:** In order to target the central nervous system, studies usually entail intravenous administration or the investigation of novel delivery method.

Other Possible Uses

- **Antidepressant Effects:** Preliminary research indicates that methylene blue may have antidepressant effects, potentially by altering neurotransmitter systems.

- **Antioxidant Properties:** Scavengers reactive oxygen species (ROS), which may be useful as a treatment in cases where oxidative stress is present.
- **Anticancer Potential:** Researched for its use in photodynamic therapy (PDT), which uses light activation to target and kill cancer cells specifically.

Diagnostics Applications of Methylene Blue

Because of its staining qualities and safety profile, methylene blue is used in a variety of diagnostic procedures across a range of medical professions. The following are a few essential diagnostic applications:

Sentinel Lymph Nodes Mapping

- **Procedure:** Sentinel lymph nodes (SLNs), the first lymph nodes to drain a tumor, are injected in the vicinity of the tumor site in order to locate and map them.
- **Indications:** Surgical oncology, mainly for breast cancer, melanoma, and other solid tumor staging and treatment planning.
- **Mechanism:** Surgeons can locate and remove these nodes for pathological evaluation because methylene blue selectively accumulates in SLNs

after being taken up by lymphatic vessels.

Identification of Gastrointestinal Fistulas and Leaks

- **Procedure:** To find leaks or fistulas in the gastrointestinal tract, methylene blue is given orally or through a nasogastric tract.
- **Indications:** Frequently used in the postoperative setting to detect leaks following gastrointestinal surgery or to discover abnormalities of the anatomy, such as fistulas.
- **Mechanism:** During imaging studies or direct visualization procedures, the dye appears at

the location of leaks or fistulas, making them visible.

Ophthalmic Staining

- **Procedure:** Stains tissues and membranes enabling easier visualization during ophthalmic surgery when applied topically or injected into the eye.
- **Indications:** Applied to enhance surgical precision and identify particular structures during procedures like vitrectomy, cataract procedures, and corneal surgeries.
- **Mechanism:** By attaching itself selectively to ocular tissues, methylene blue improves contrast and helps surgeons in

delicate maneuvers within the eye.

Urology Diagnostic Tool

- **Procedure:** Intravenous injection used in urological procedures to evaluate renal function and identify anomalies in the urine.
- **Indications:** Applied in research on renal blood flow assessment, ureteral patency evaluation, and urine leak identification.
- **Mechanism:** The kidneys expel the dye, which makes it possible to visualize urine flow and identify anomalies in the urinary tract.

Histological and Microbiological Studies Staining

- **Procedure:** Stain cells, tissues, and microorganism for microscopic examination in laboratory settings.
- **Indications:** Crucial for recognizing microbial infections, abnormal tissue, and cellular structures in histopathology.
- **Mechanism:** Methylene blue gives contrast and improves visualization under a microscope by binding to proteins and nucleic acids.

Dermatology Visualization

- **Procedure:** Applied topically or intravenously to assist in the identification and management of skin disorders.

- **Indications:** Helps define the delineation of lesion; assess skin perfusion, and direct treatments such as skin biopsies.
- **Mechanism:** Facilitates accurate diagnosis and treatment planning by defining tissue boundaries and enhancing contrast.

Assessment in Veterinary Medicine

- **Procedure:** Used in veterinary diagnostics for a number of purposes, including as surgical mapping, urological studies, and wound assessment.

- **Indications:** Tissue staining for surgical guidance, gastrointestinal leakage, and lymphatic drainage patterns are all detected using indications similar to those in human medicine.
- **Mechanism:** Improves visualization of animal clinical states and anatomical structures by utilizing the dye's staining properties.

Possible Future Application for Methylene Blue

Beyond its current medical and industrial applications, methylene blue, known for its varied properties and historical uses, is still being researched for prospective uses. The following are some new fields where methylene blue might be used in the future:

Antiviral Treatment

- **Mechanism:** Studies suggest that methylene blue might have antiviral properties by preventing viruses from replicating or entering host cells.
- **Potential Applications:** Its effectiveness against a variety of viruses, such as coronaviruses like SARS-CoV-2, herpes simplex virus (HSV), and HIV, is being researched.
- **Advantages:** In cases of drug-resistant strains or newly emerging viral outbreaks, this

could offer an alternate or supplemental treatment option for viral infections.

Neuroprotection and Improving Cognitive Function

- **Mechanism:** Methylene blue improves mitochondrial function, lowers oxidative stress, and increases neuroplasticity, which may help with cognitive function and neurodegenerative disorders.
- **Potential Applications:** Investigated for the treatment of ailments such as traumatic brain injury (TBI), Parkinson's disease, Alzheimer's disease, and age-related cognitive decline.

- **Advantages:** Provides neuroprotective effects that may slow the progression of disease, promote general brain health, and improve cognitive outcomes.

Photodynamic Therapy (PDT) for cancer

- **Mechanism:** When light is activated in photodynamic therapy (PDT), methylene blue produces reactive oxygen species (ROS) that specifically target and kill cancer cells.
- **Potential Applications:** Extending its application in oncology to treat a wider range of cancers, such as solid

tumors, bladder cancer, and superficial skin cancers.
- **Advantages:** Offers the possibility of combination therapies together with a targeted treatment strategy that has fewer systemic side effects than traditional chemotherapy.

Healing Wounds and Tissue Repair

- **Mechanism:** By reducing inflammation, preventing infections, and boosting tissue regeneration, methylene blue's antioxidant and antimicrobial qualities may aid in the healing of wounds.
- **Potential Applications:** Being researched for application in

skin graft surgeries, surgical incision healing, and chronic wound care.

- **Advantages:** May quicken the healing process, raise the percentage of wound closure, and lessen complications brought on by non-healing wounds.

Antioxidant Therapy

- **Mechanism:** scavenges reactive oxygen species (ROS) to shield cells from oxidative damage linked to inflammation, aging, and a host of diseases.
- **Potential Applications:** Explored for ailments like cardiovascular disease, complications from diabetes,

and inflammatory disorders where oxidative stress is a significant factor.
- **Advantages:** May be used therapeutically to reduce damage caused by oxidative stress while maintaining tissue integrity and cellular function.

Remediation of the Environment

- **Mechanism:** Because it can identify and interact with pollutants in soil and water, it is used in environmental monitoring and remediation projects.
- **Potential Applications:** Applied in the identification and degradation of pollutants, water

quality monitoring, and the encouragement of environmentally sustainable practices.

- **Advantages:** Promotes ecological health and human well-being while helping with pollution identification and cleaning, which contributes to environmental conservation.

Pharmacokinetics and Pharmacodynamics of Methylene Blue

Pharmacokinetics

- **Absorption:**

Oral Administration: The gastrointestinal tract readily absorbs methylene blue, but the liver extensively first-pass metabolizes it.

Intravenous Administration: Provides quick and thorough systemic distribution.

- **Distribution:**

Tissue Distribution: Methylene blue is extensively distributed throughout the body, especially in well vascularized tissues.

Blood-Brain Barrier (BBB): The BBB is somewhat penetrated, allowing effects on the central nervous system.

- **Metabolism:**

Liver Metabolism: NADPH-dependent reductases mainly

metabolize leukomethylene blue in the liver to produce the reduced form of the substance.

Half-Life: Varying, usually between 4 to 6 hours in adults, dependent on renal clearance, age, and liver function, among other factors.

- **Excretion:**

Renal Excretion: Mostly excreted in urine unchanged.

Biliary Excretion: Bile excretes a small portion.

Pharmacodynamics

- **Mechanism of Action:**

Redox Properties: Functions as a redox agent, regulating cellular redox reactions by accepting and giving away electrons.

Enzyme Inhibition: Affects the metabolism of neurotransmitters by inhibiting enzymes such as monoamine oxidase (MAO).

Nucleic Acid Binding: Binds to proteins, nucleic acids (DNA, RNA), other cellular components and affecting cellular processes.

Impact on Hemoglobin:

- **Methemoglobin Reduction:** Accepts electrons from NADPH-methemoglobin reductase to transform methemoglobin back into functional hemoglobin.

Neurological Effects:

- **Neuroprotective:** May be helpful in neurodegenerative diseases, improves mitochondrial function, lowers oxidative stress, and modifies neurotransmitter systems.

Antimicrobial and Antiparasitic Effects:

- **Mechanism:** Affects the survival of bacteria and parasites by disrupting microbial membranes, inhibiting vital enzymes, and producing reactive oxygen species (ROS) when exposed to light.

Clinical Effects:

- **Antimalarial:** Blocks heme polymerase and interferes with the metabolism of parasites by selectively accumulating in red blood cells infected with Plasmodium.
- **Antidepressant:** May have antidepressant effects through modifying the levels of neurotransmitters, especially serotonin and norepinephrine.

Clinical Considerations

Dosage and Administration:

- **Methemoglobinemia:** Based on the patient's age, weight, and degree of methemoglobinemia, an intravenous 1% solution is administered at doses that are adjusted.
- **Diagnostic Uses:** Depending on the process and intended application, administered topically or intravenously.

Adverse Effects:

- **Methemoglobinemia:** May have negative effects, especially after long-term use or high doses.

- **Effects on the Central Nervous System:** In rare cases, may result in headache, dizziness, or disorientation.
- **Gastrointestinal Effects:** In rare instances, nausea, vomiting, and stomach pain have been recorded.

Drug Interactions:

- **MAO Inhibitors:** Adverse effects may be amplified when used concurrently with other MAO inhibitors.
- **Antidepressants:** Possible interactions between other antidepressants and selective serotonin reuptake inhibitors (SSRIs) that impact serotonin levels.

Future Directions

- **Research:** Ongoing studies investigate novel therapeutic applications, including cancer treatments, neuroprotection, and antiviral therapies.
- **Clinical Innovation:** Creating targeted delivery methods to maximize efficacy and minimize side effects.
- **Environmental Applications:** Increasing involvement in environmental cleanup and monitoring efforts.

Methylene blue's pharmacokinetics and pharmacodynamics can be used to better understand clinical applications, possible advantages, and considerations for safe and efficient administration for both clinical practice and research.

Chapter Five

The Hazards and Side Effects of Methylene Blue

Despite being widely regarded as safe when used correctly and under medical supervision, methylene blue may have adverse effects, particularly when used in high doses or for a prolonged period of time. The following are the considerations regarding its toxicity and adverse effects.

Common Side Effects

- **Mild Gastrointestinal Symptoms:**

Description: Higher doses or oral administration may result in nausea, vomiting, and abdominal pain.

Management: Supportive care or dose adjustments can be used to address symptoms, which usually are self-limiting.

- **Exploration of Urine and Feces:**

Description: Methylene blue is a safe dye that can give urine and feces a blue or green color, although it may be alarming to patients.

Explanation: The excretion of unchanged methylene blue and its metabolites is what causes this discoloration.

Rare but Serious Side Effects

- **Methemoglobinemia:**

Description: Despite being employed as a treatment for the condition, high dosages of methylene blue have the paradoxical ability to cause or worsen methemoglobinemia.

Mechanism: Hemoglobin's ability to carry oxygen can be reduced when it is oxidized to methemoglobin at high methylene blue concentrations.

Symptoms: dyspnea, possibly life-threatening hypoxia, and cyanosis (blue coloring of the skin and mucous membranes).

Management: In severe cases, promptly identify the condition and administer methylene blue antidote treatment.

- **Serotonin Syndrome:**

Description: Methylene blue may trigger serotonin syndrome in those who are predisposed or when taken in conjunction with serotonergics medicines.

Mechanism: Potentiates the effects of serotonin by inhibiting its reuptake, which can cause symptoms like tremor, agitation, hyperthermia, and altered mental status.

Management: Immediate discontinuation and supportive

treatment, such as benzodiazepines for agitation and cooling techniques for hyperthermia.

- **Impact on the Central Nervous System:**

Description: In rare cases, methylene blue may result in neurological symptoms such tremors, headaches, dizziness, and confusion.

Mechanism: Its neurotransmitter-modulating qualities may have possible CNS effects, especially at higher doses or in sensitive people.

Management: When the dosage of methylene blue is reduced or stopped, the symptoms usually go away.

Precautions and Contraindications

- **Insufficiency of glucose-6-phosphate dehydrogenase (G6PD):**

Risk: When exposed to methylene blue, people with G6PD deficiency have a higher chance of developing methemoglobinemia.

Explanation: A G6PD deficit affects the body's capacity to produce enough NADPH, which is necessary for the conversion of methemoglobin back into hemoglobin.

Screening: Prior to administering methylene blue, screening for G6PD deficiency is advised, particularly in areas where this genetic disorder is highly prevalent.

- **Reaction with Inhibitors of MAO:**

Risk: Serotonin syndrome can result from using methylene blue concurrently with monoamine oxidase inhibitors (MAOIs) or within two weeks after stopping MAOIs.

Explanation: By inhibiting serotonin metabolism, methylene blue and MAOIs can both lead to excessive serotonin buildup.

Avoidance: When taking these drugs at the same time, careful consideration and monitoring are required.

Environmental Consideration

- **Toxicology in Water:**

Risk: When released into natural water bodies or in large amounts, methylene blue can be toxic to aquatic life.

Precautions: In order to reduce the influence on the environment, wastewater treatment and proper disposal are essential.

Studies of Clinical Cases

I don't have access to patient information or particular clinical case studies. If it would be useful, I can, however, offer fictitious instances or go over basic circumstances pertaining to the clinical application of methylene blue. For example, we may talk about a fictitious situation when methylene blue is administered for methemoglobinemia or when it's used as a diagnostic tool during surgery. Tell me how you would like to continue!

Reviewing Clinical Trials

Of course! Methylene blue's effectiveness and safety have been investigated in clinical trials for a range of medical conditions. The following summarizes significant clinical trials and their findings:

Chapter Six

Overview of Clinical Trials

- **Methemoglobinemia and Methylene Blue:**

Study Objective: Determine if methylene blue is useful in treating methemoglobinemia, a disorder in which hemoglobin is degraded and unable to bind oxygen efficiently.

Findings: Clinical trials have regularly shown that administering methylene blue intravenously can quickly and effectively lower methemoglobin levels. In cases of severe methemoglobinemia, it is regarded as a first-line therapy.

- **Diagnostic Applications in Surgery:**

Study Objective: Assess the application of methylene blue as a diagnostic tool in different surgical operations, such as cancer surgery sentinel lymph node identification.

Findings: Studies have shown that methylene blue efficiently stains lymphatic tissue, assisting surgeons in accurately identifying and removing lymph nodes during procedures such as melanoma excision and breast cancer surgery.

- **Antidepressant Effects:**

Study Objective: Examine Methylene Blue's possible antidepressant properties, especially in cases of treatment-resistant depression.

Findings: Research indicates that methylene blue at low dosages may have antidepressant effects through improving the activity of monoamine neurotransmitters and lowering oxidative stress. Although the results are encouraging, more investigation is needed to determine the product's safety and effectiveness in clinical settings.

- **Neuroprotective Effects:**

Study Objective: Examine the possible neuroprotective benefits of methylene blue in the treatment of traumatic brain damage and neurodegenerative illnesses.

Findings: By enhancing mitochondrial function and reducing oxidative stress, methylene blue may mitigate neuronal damage, according to preliminary trials. To validate these findings and establish the best dosage and treatment regimens, larger-scale research is required.

- **Photodynamic Therapy (PDT):**

Study Objective: Evaluate methylene blue's effectiveness in photodynamic therapy for a range of cancers, such as bladder and skin cancers.

Findings: Clinical studies have shown that methylene blue can specifically target and kill cancer cells while preserving healthy tissue when it is exposed to light. Comparing PDT with methylene blue to conventional chemotherapy, the former shows potential as a localized treatment approach with less systemic side effects.

Uses in Various Industries

Methylene blue was first created as a synthetic dye for the textile industry, but it has since found a wide range of uses in other industries as well. The following are some important sectors that use methylene blue:

Textile Sector

- **Dyeing and coloration:**

Application: Methylene blue is a dye used in the textile industry to give fabrics a rich blue hue.

Advantages: Offers versatility and colorfastness for dyeing both natural and synthetic textiles.

Healthcare and Medical Sectors

- **Medicine:**

Treatment for Methemoglobinemia: Intravenous injections are used to restore hemoglobin's ability to carry oxygen.

Diagnostic Tool: Used during surgery to detect sentinel lymph nodes and visualize lymphatic drainage.

Antidepressant Therapy: Investigated for possible antidepressant effects, especially in cases of depression that is resistant to therapy.

- **Photodynamic therapy (PDT):**

Application: Methylene blue, which is activated by light, is used in PDT to target and kill cancer cells specifically in skin and bladder cancers.

Applications in the Environment

- **Water and Environmental Monitoring:**

Pollutant Detection: It use as tracer dye to detect leaks in plumbing and industrial pipelines.

Water Quality Testing: Used in environmental research to assess pollution levels and monitor water quality.

Investigation and Lab Applications

- **Biological Staining:**

Microscopy: Tissues, cells, and microorganism are stained for microscopic examination in histology and microbiology.

Cell Biology Research: Facilitates the scientific visualization of cellular processes and structures.

Additional Industrial Uses

- **Photography:**

Toning Agent: Historically used as a toning agent to improve picture stability and contrast in black-and-white photography.

Electronics:

Electrochemical Applications: Because of its redox properties, it is used in electrochemical cells and sensors.

Future Prospects

- **Antiviral and Antimicrobial usage:**

Research: investigated for antimicrobial usage in infection control as well as possible antiviral qualities against viruses such as HIV and SARS-CoV-2.

Implications of Methylene Blue for the Environment

Methylene blue is useful in many industrial and medical applications, but because of its possible toxicity and persistence, it presents environmental concerns. An outline of its effects on the environment is provided below:

Toxicology of Water

- **Effect on Aquatic Organism:**

Toxicity: Fish and other aquatic organism are especially vulnerable to the negative effects of methylene blue.

Exposure Route: Wastewater from hospitals or industrial activities discharged into water bodies.

Negative Effects: May build up in tissues and interfere with respiratory functions, which can be detrimental to the health of aquatic ecosystems.

Persistence and Biodegradation

- **Environmental Persistence:**

Chemical Stability: Methylene blue has a comparatively stable chemical makeup and can withstand prolonged exposure to the environment.

Degradation: Environmental factors such as pH, temperature, and microbial activity affect the rate at which materials biodegrade.

Bioaccumulation: May accumulate in organism through the food chain, increasing the danger of long-term exposure.

Treatment of Wastewater

- **Treatment Challenges:**

Removal Efficiency: Because of the chemical properties of methylene blue, conventional wastewater treatment methods may not be able to remove it completely.

Secondary Pollution: Ecological effects and secondary pollution may result from residual methylene blue discharged into water bodies.

Management and Regulatory Practices

- **Environmental Regulations:**

Monitoring and Limitations: In order to safeguard aquatic ecosystems, regulations are in place in some areas with particular discharge limitations.

Best Practices: Promotes the use of best management practices in the handling, treatment, and disposal of waste containing methylene blue in industry and healthcare facilities.

Strategies for Mitigation

Environmental Management:

- **Waste Minimization:** Encourages the use of chemicals and dyes that have less of an impact on the environment.

Advanced Treatment Technologies: Investigating and implementing advance techniques to improve methylene blue removal wastewater.

Conclusion

Methylene blue is a versatile compound with a wide range of uses in various disciplines and industries. It was first used as a synthetic dye in textiles, but it has since developed into a vital instrument for environmental monitoring, research, and medicine.

Methylene blue plays a vital role in medicine, helping with surgical procedures for lymph node mapping, treating methemoglobinemia, and maybe providing therapeutic benefits in oncology and neurology. It is adaptable in a variety of diagnostic and therapeutic applications due to its special qualities as a redox agent and its capacity to interact with biological components.

Methylene blue has uses in medicine as well as environmental monitoring and remediation, though due to its potential toxicity to aquatic life, handling and disposal practices must be done carefully.

In the future, methylene blue's usage will be further explored and improved upon by ongoing study, underscoring its ongoing significance and potential in tackling present and emerging issues in science, health, and environmental sustainability.

Methylene blue is still a useful tool in modern industry and medicine, despite its negative effects on the environment. Future advancements and improvements in this field are anticipated.

www.ingramcontent.com/pod-product-compliance
Lightning Source LLC
Chambersburg PA
CBHW070152230526
45471CB00002B/623